I0070861

Sharing Hearts to Art:
The Journey

A Storybook for Children and Adolescents
Who Experienced Abuse or Neglect

Alexandra Schick, MD
Illustrated by Kathi Dery

This book is dedicated to all the children and adolescents who so beautifully drew their broken hearts. By offering their drawings, they were hoping to help and teach others who may also have been abused or neglected. Many have been touched by their courage to open their hearts and by their dedication to be of service in the process. I thank them for inspiring the creation of this book. I also thank Margaret Heasley for her friendly support and her wise guidance. Finally, I thank Kathi Dery for her beautiful artwork and for her ability to reach children's hearts with her drawings.

Alexandra Schick, MD, Child and Adolescent Psychiatrist

"When the heart listens, angels sing."

Anonymous

This storybook is for children and adolescents who have a history of abuse or neglect. It seeks to teach them some common core feelings and defenses that can happen in such a situation. It also seeks to teach them the about some of the help that they can receive. A youth who has experienced abuse and neglect will often tend to be withdrawn and isolated. We are hoping that this storybook will help them realize that they are not alone feeling this way and that they are worthy of getting help. We also hope that it will encourage them to open up and reach out. Workbooks will be available to complete the storybook so that mental health professionals may further work with the youth in therapy using a similar approach.

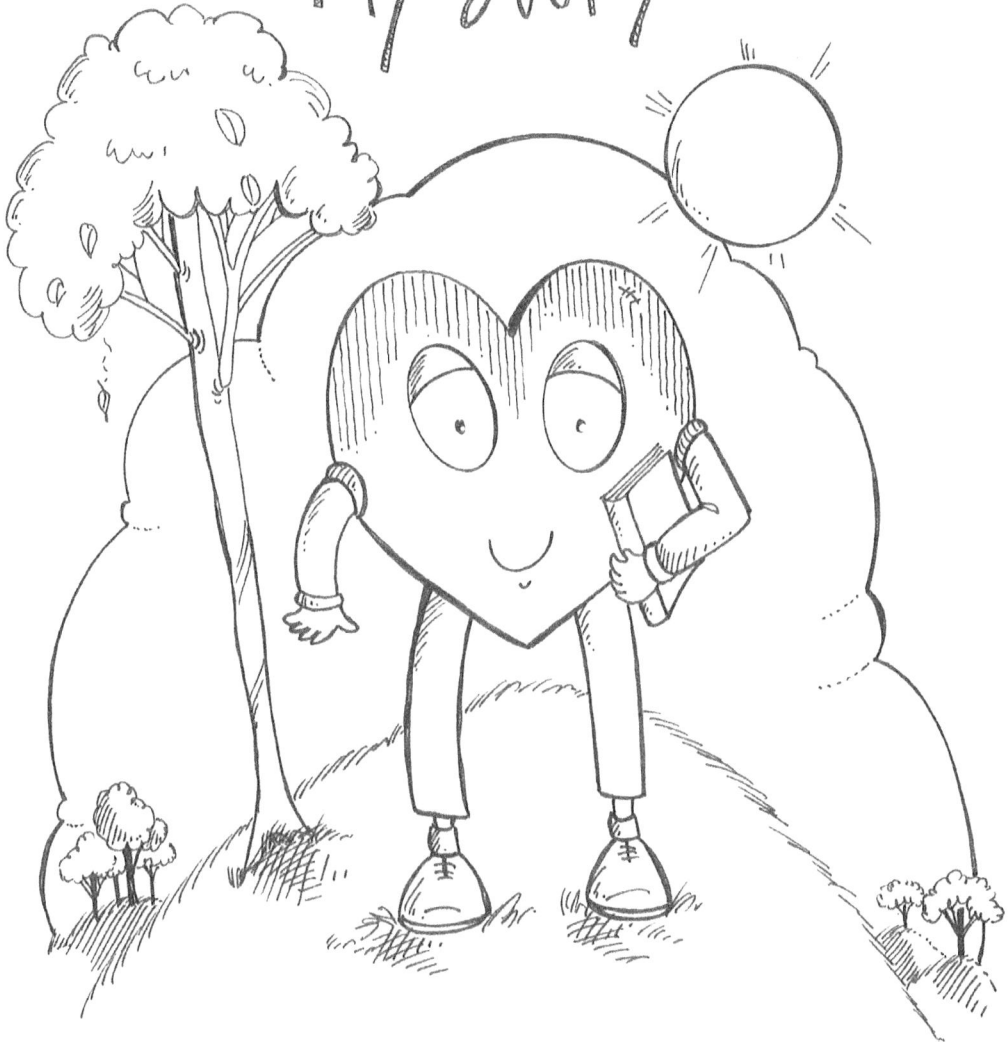

When I was young I was broken.

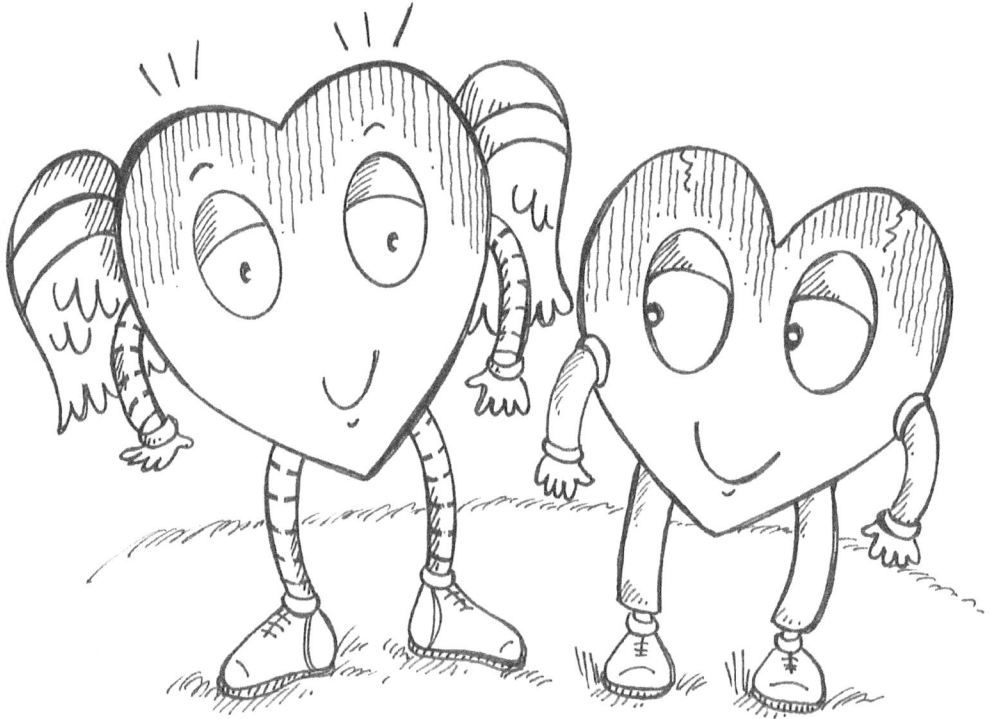

I met a helper heart who guided me along the way.

I am sharing my story with you to teach you about your heart and to encourage you to get help.

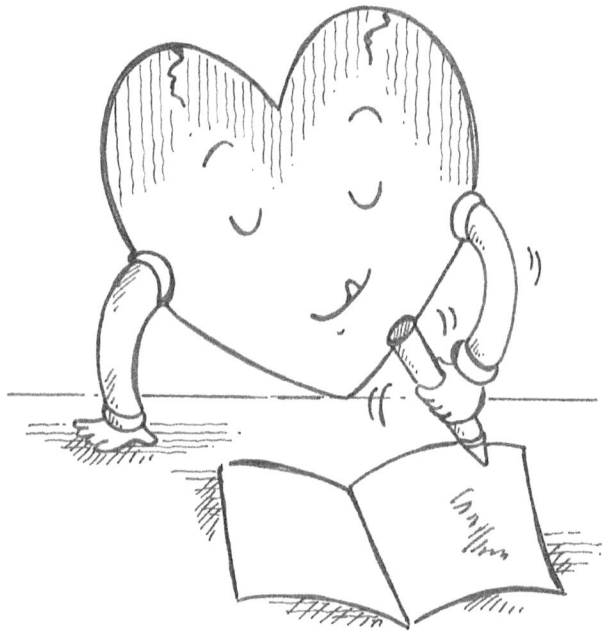

you can color the drawings that you relate to if you want.

When I was young I got
hurt and I went
through
many hardships.

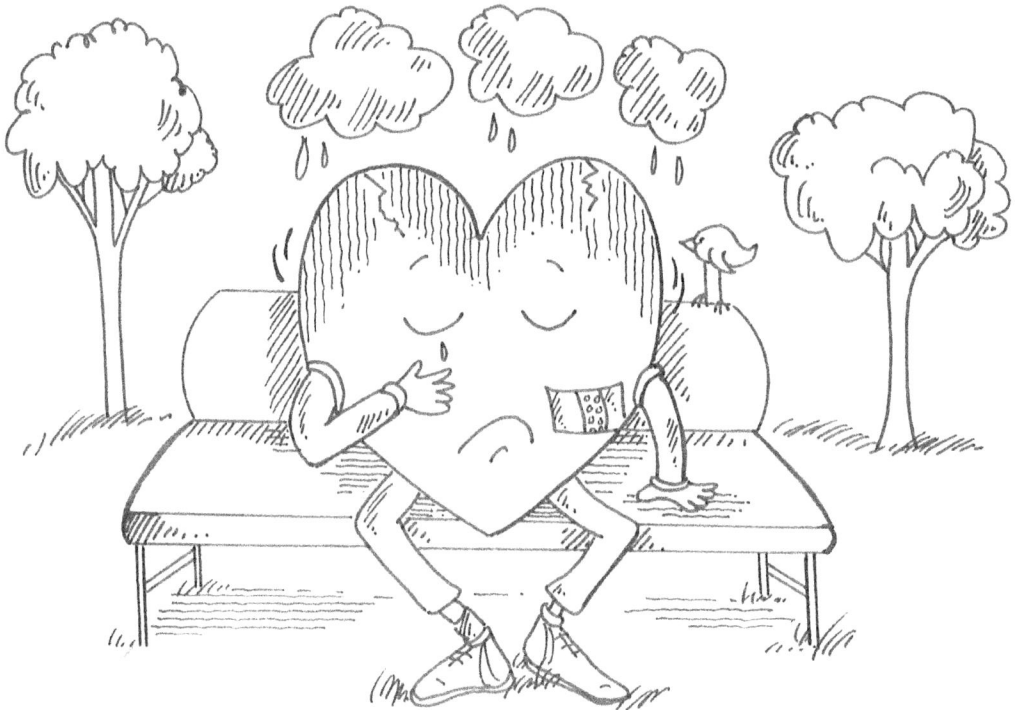

It made me feel broken.

As my life turned
upside down,

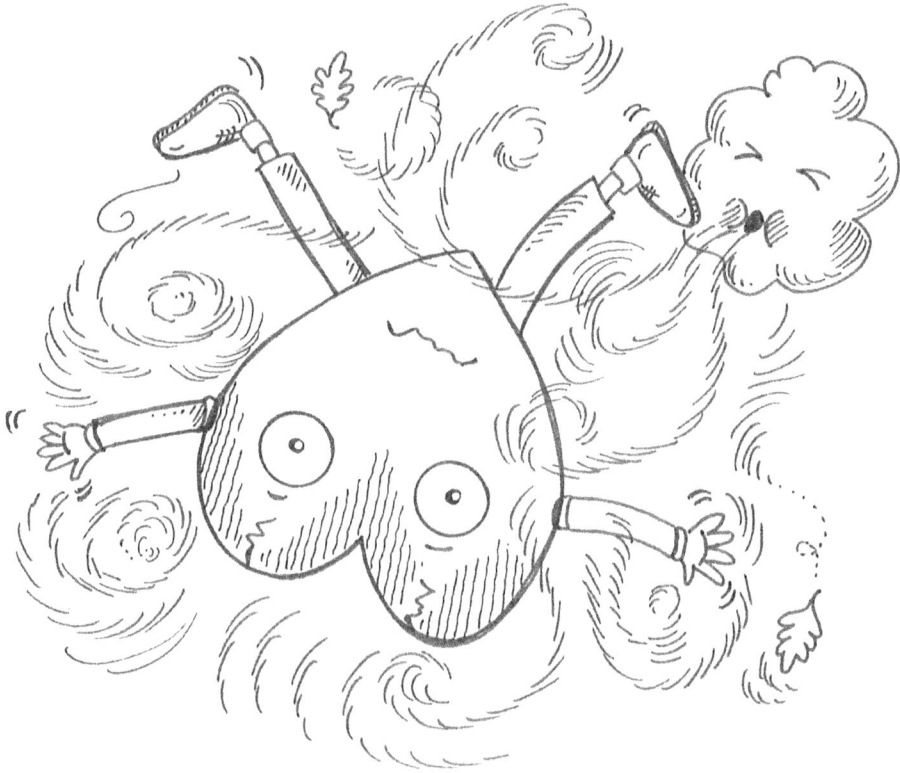

I also felt that I was
turned upside
down
as well.

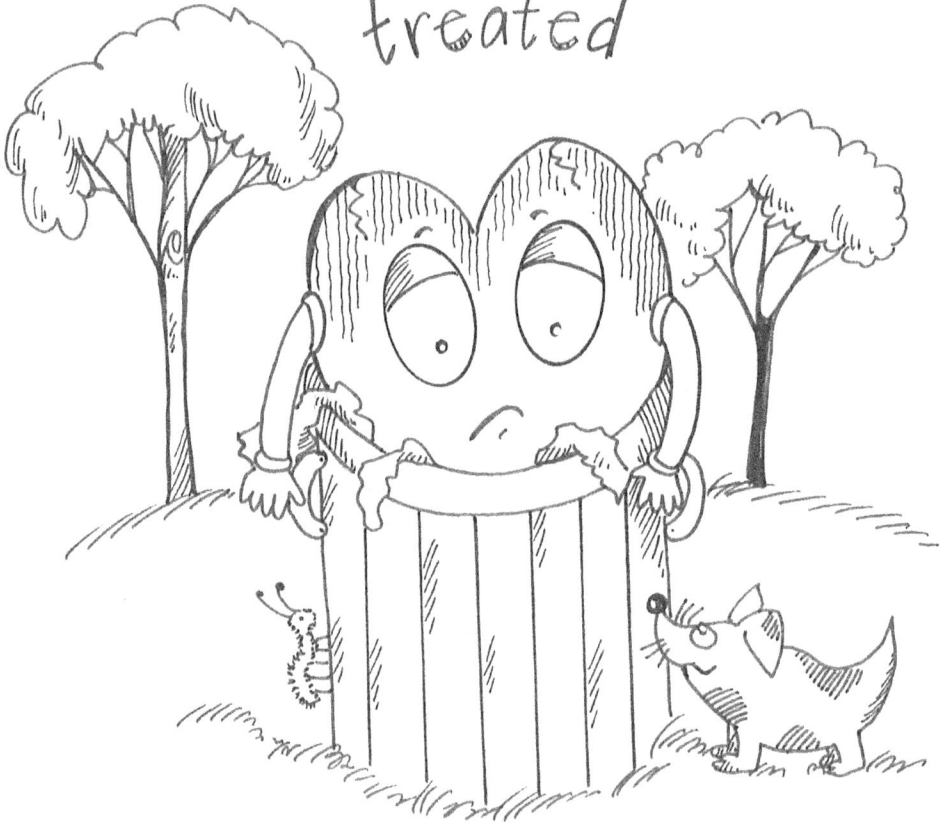

The way I was treated

made me believe that
I was
not worth much.

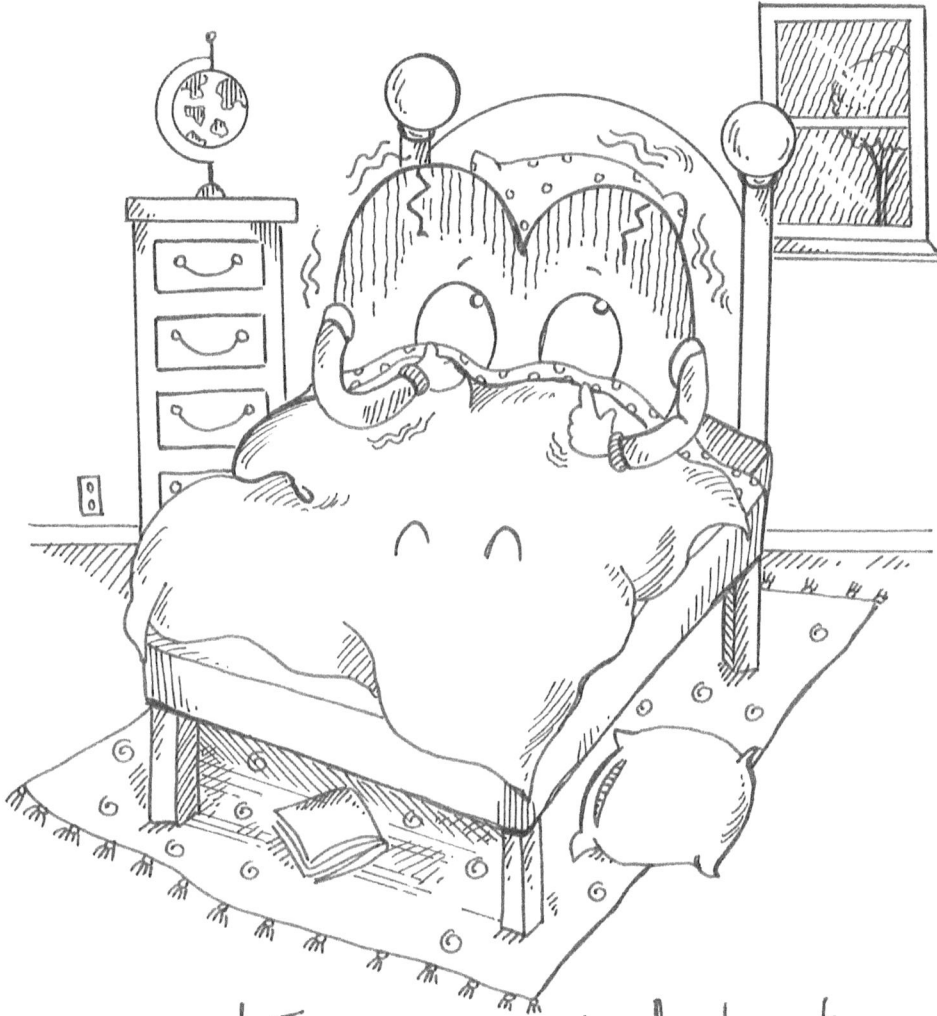

I was scared. I was anxious about my past,

and I was worried about my future.

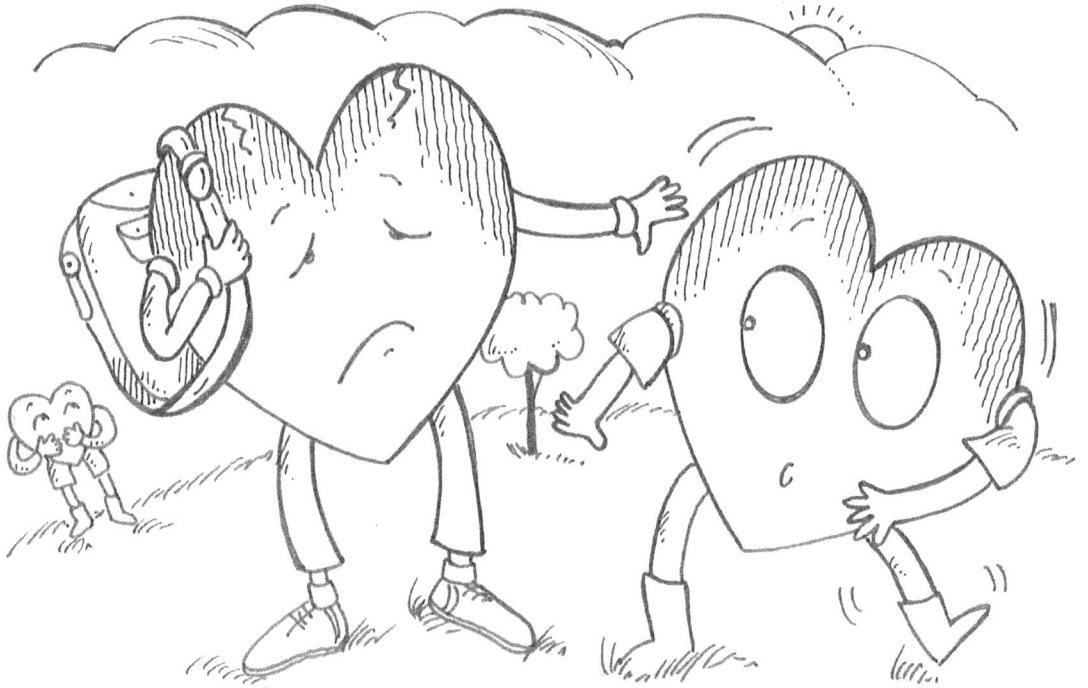

I had a harder time trusting others.

I even wanted to push people away at times.

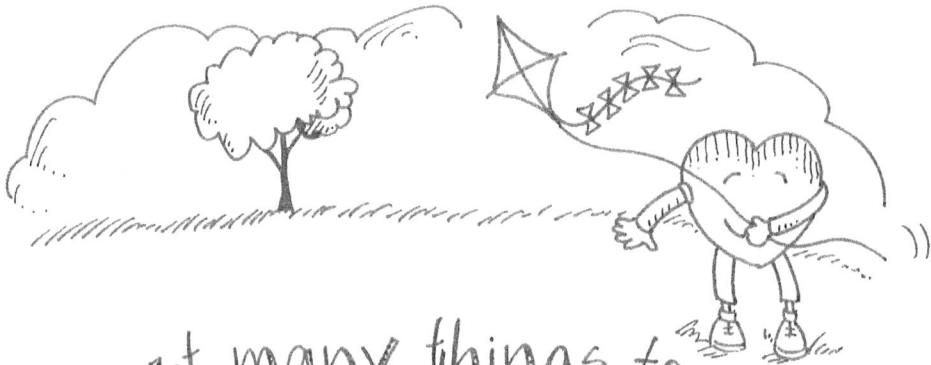

I kept many things to myself.

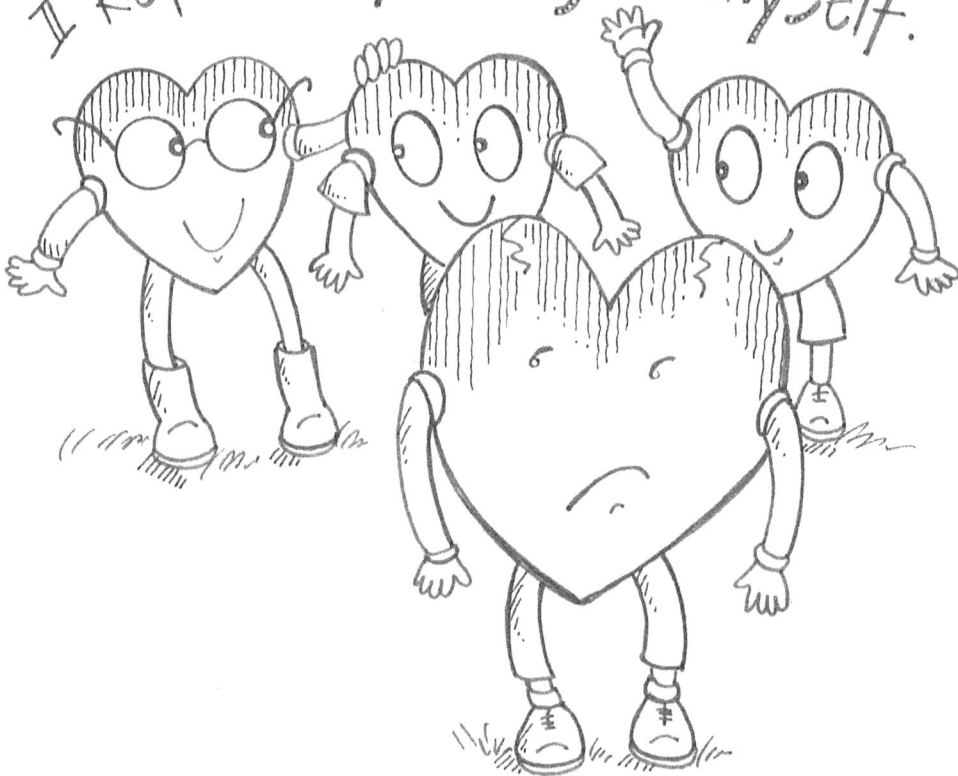

I felt that others would not
understand me and that
I was different.

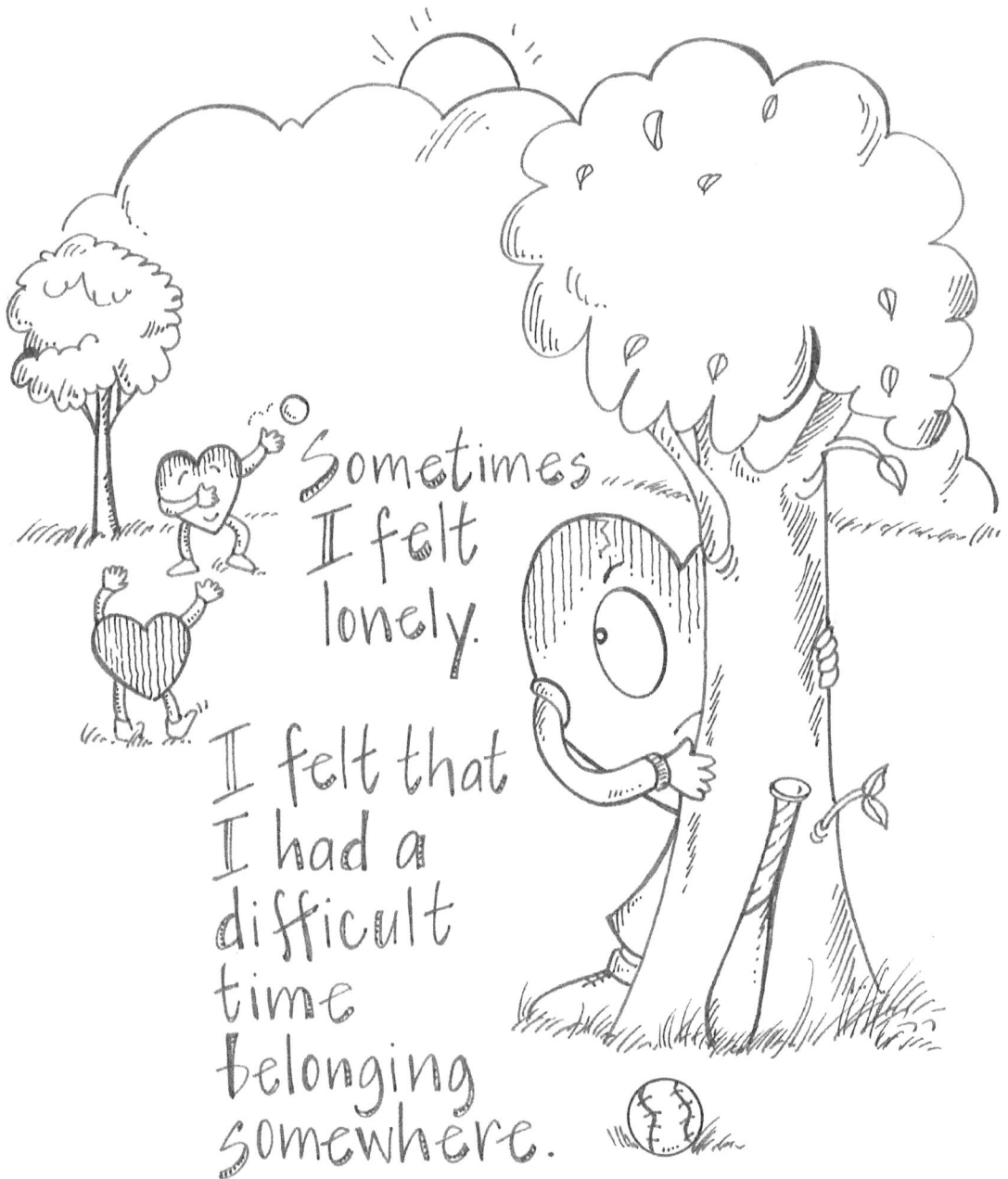

Sometimes I felt lonely.

I felt that I had a difficult time belonging somewhere.

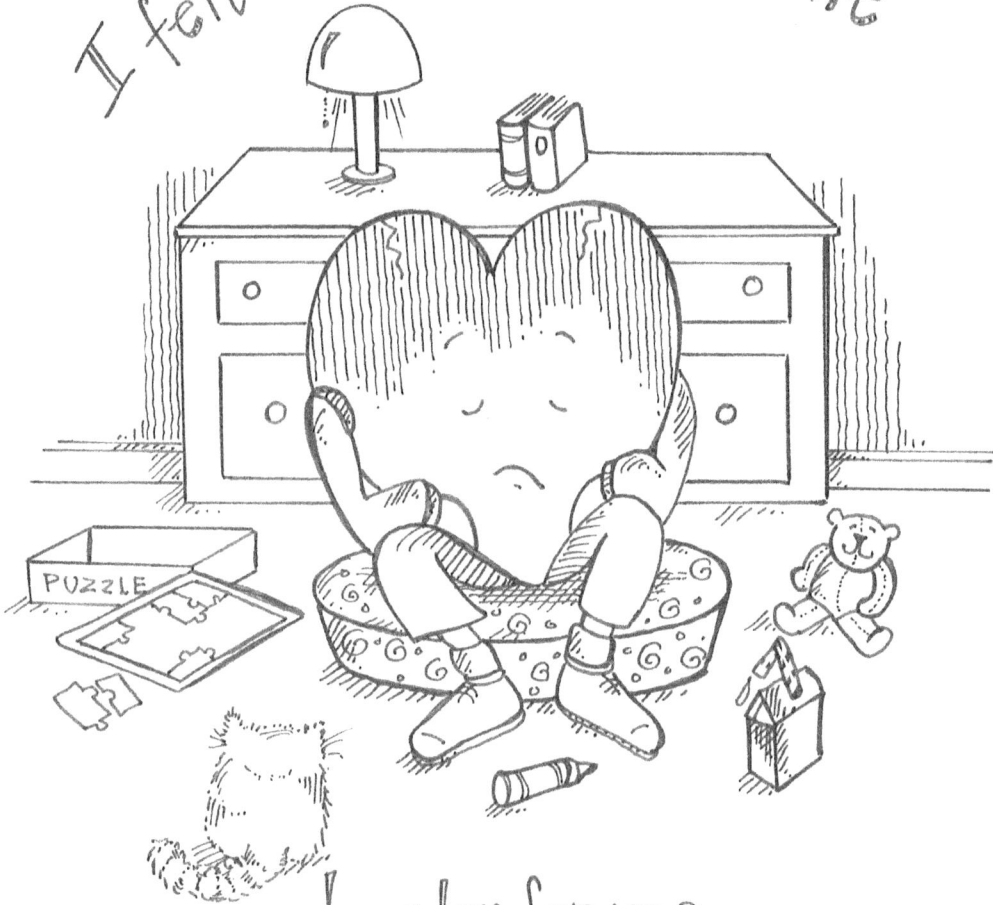

I was sad.
I felt heavy and it became

harder for me
to
have fun.

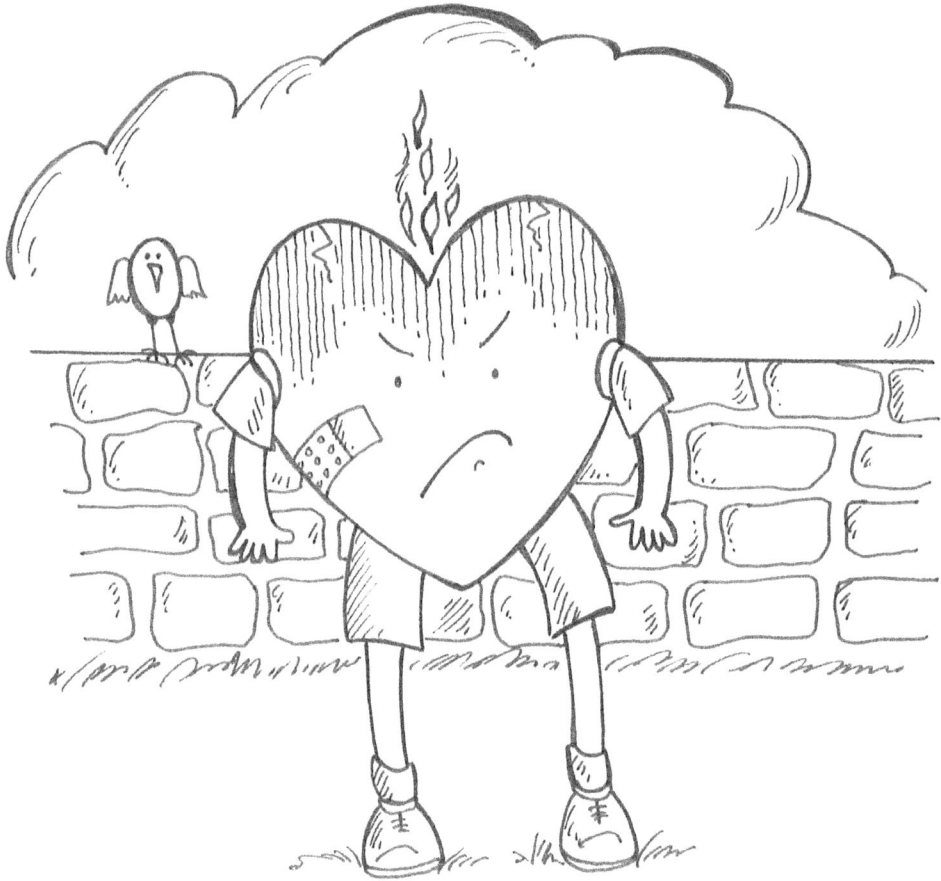

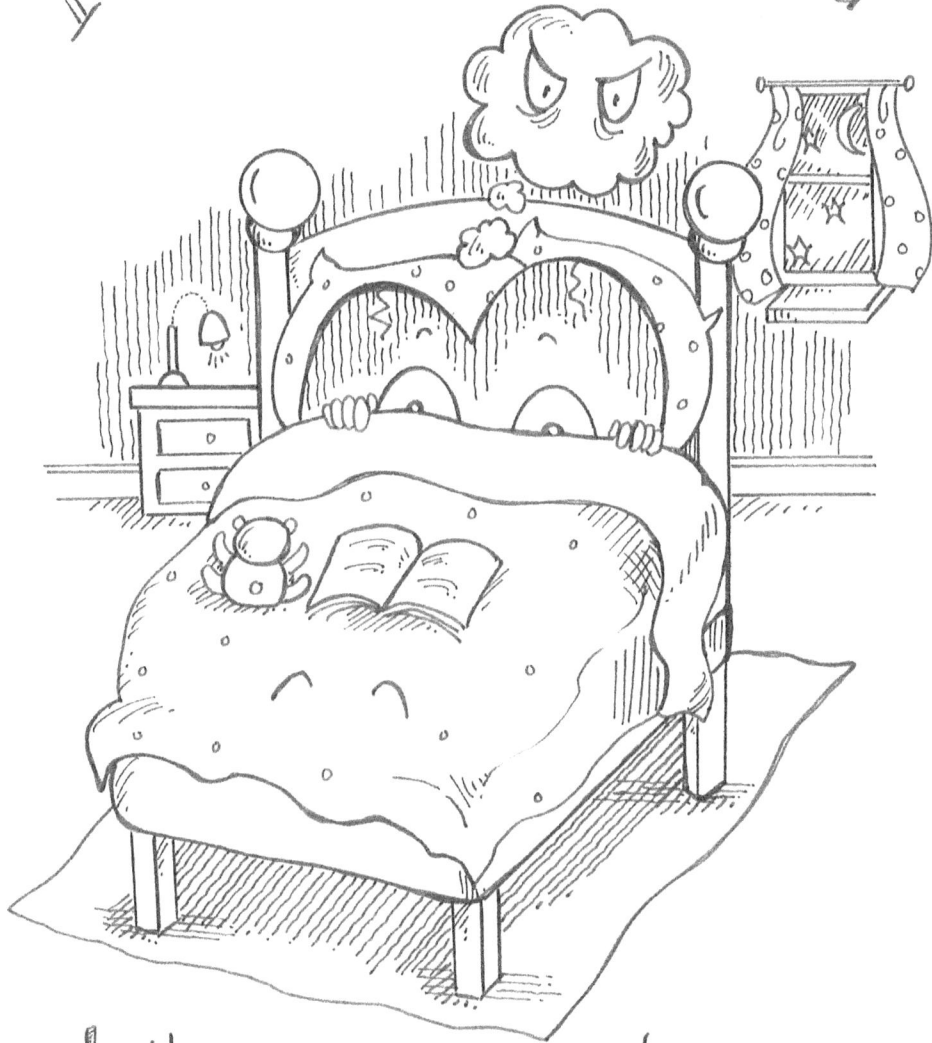

I had bad memories and bad dreams

bothering me sometimes.

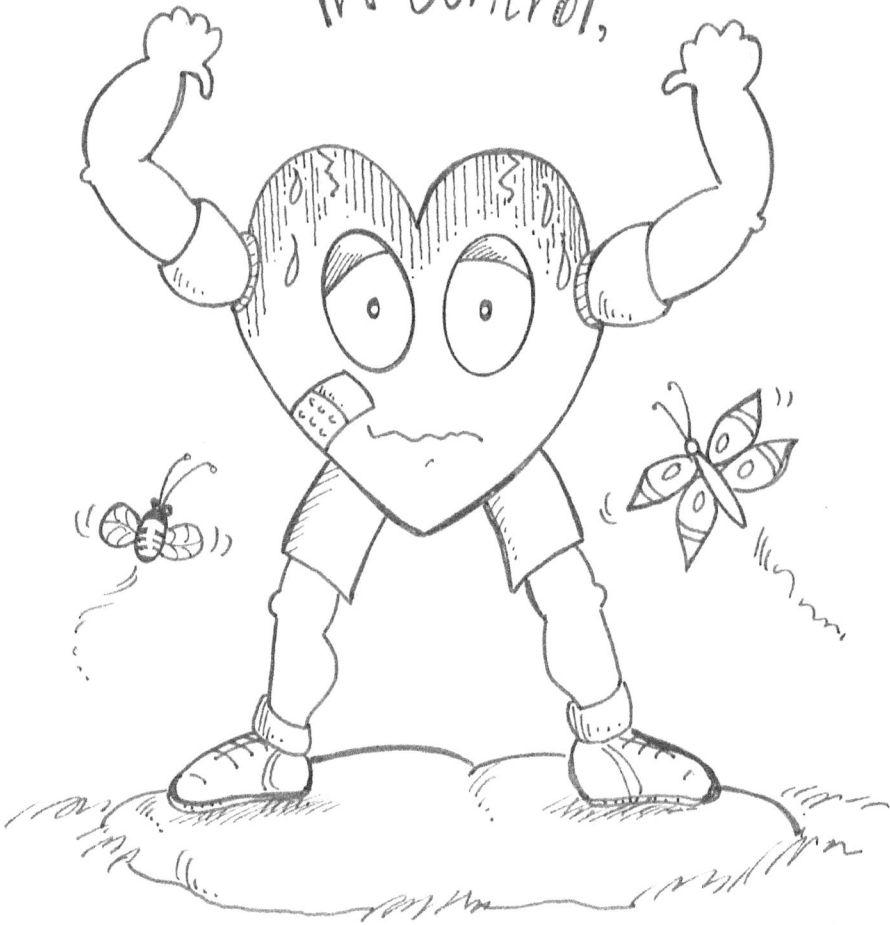

I put on
a mask
and hid

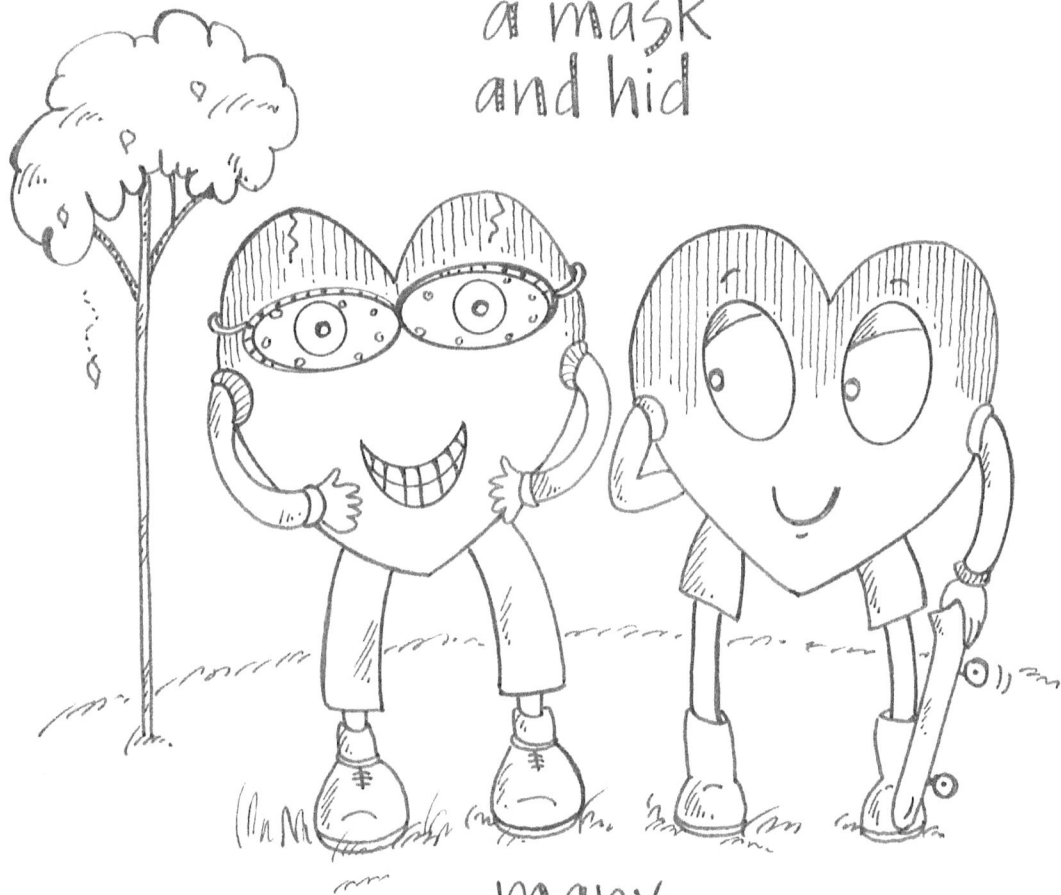

many
of my
feelings.

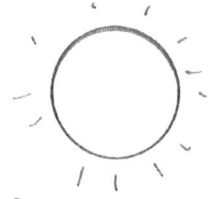

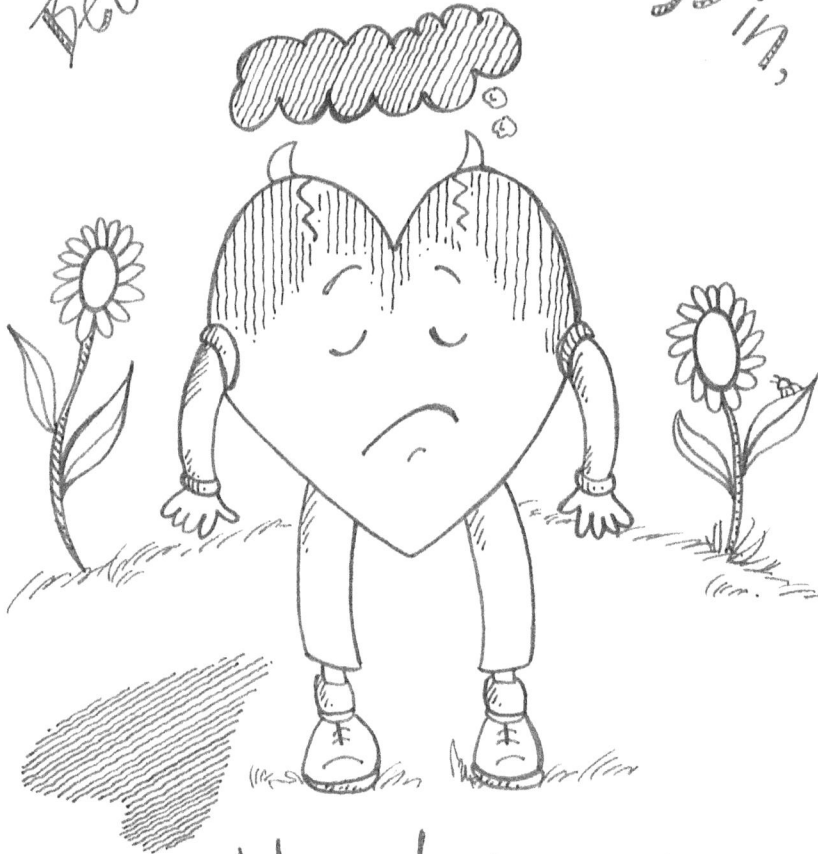

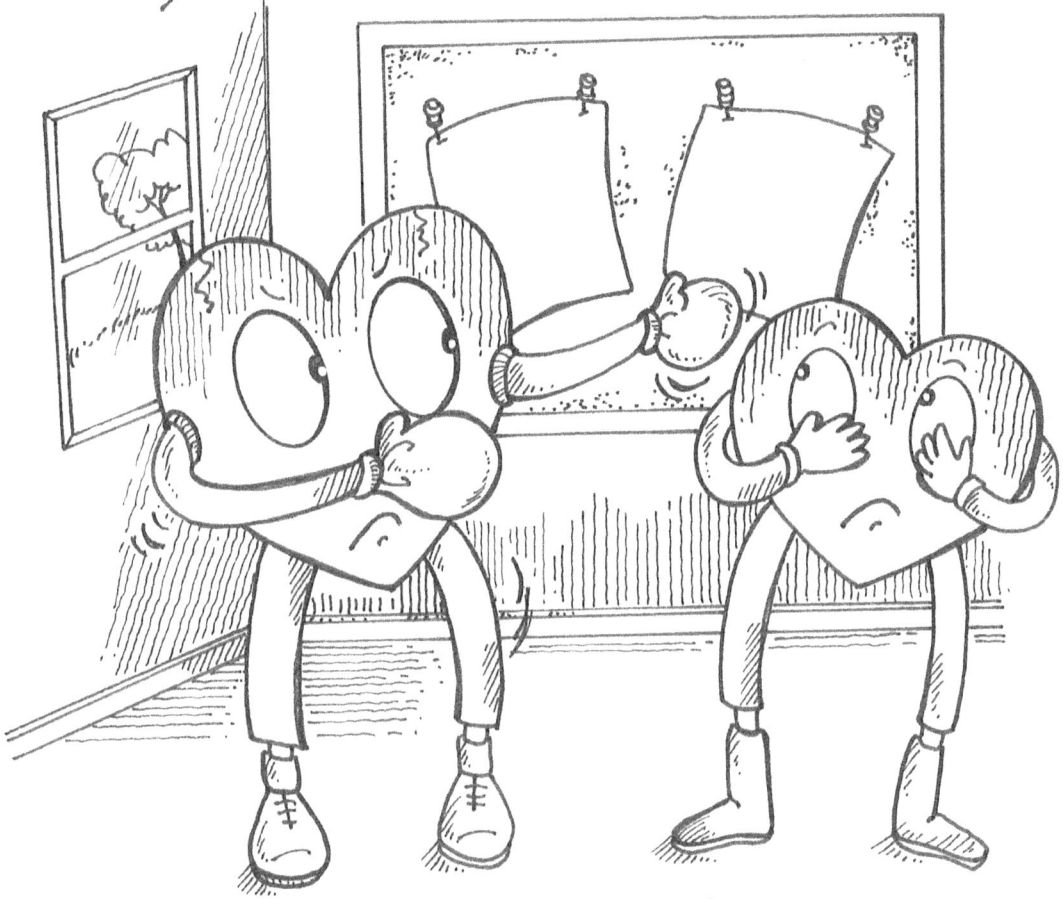

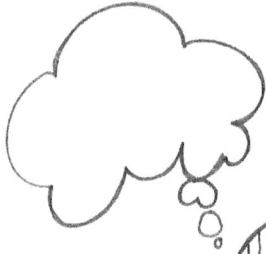

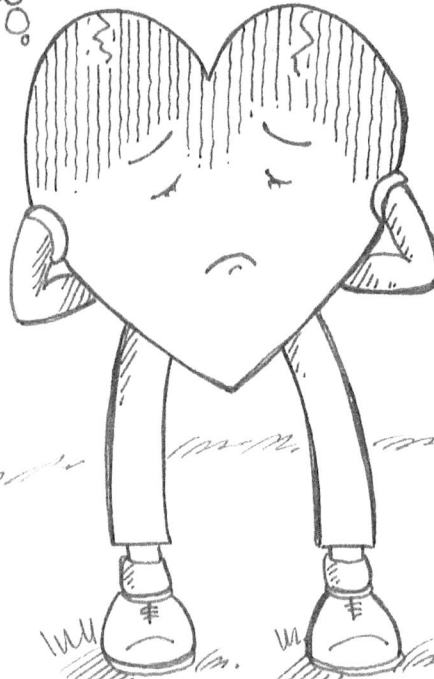

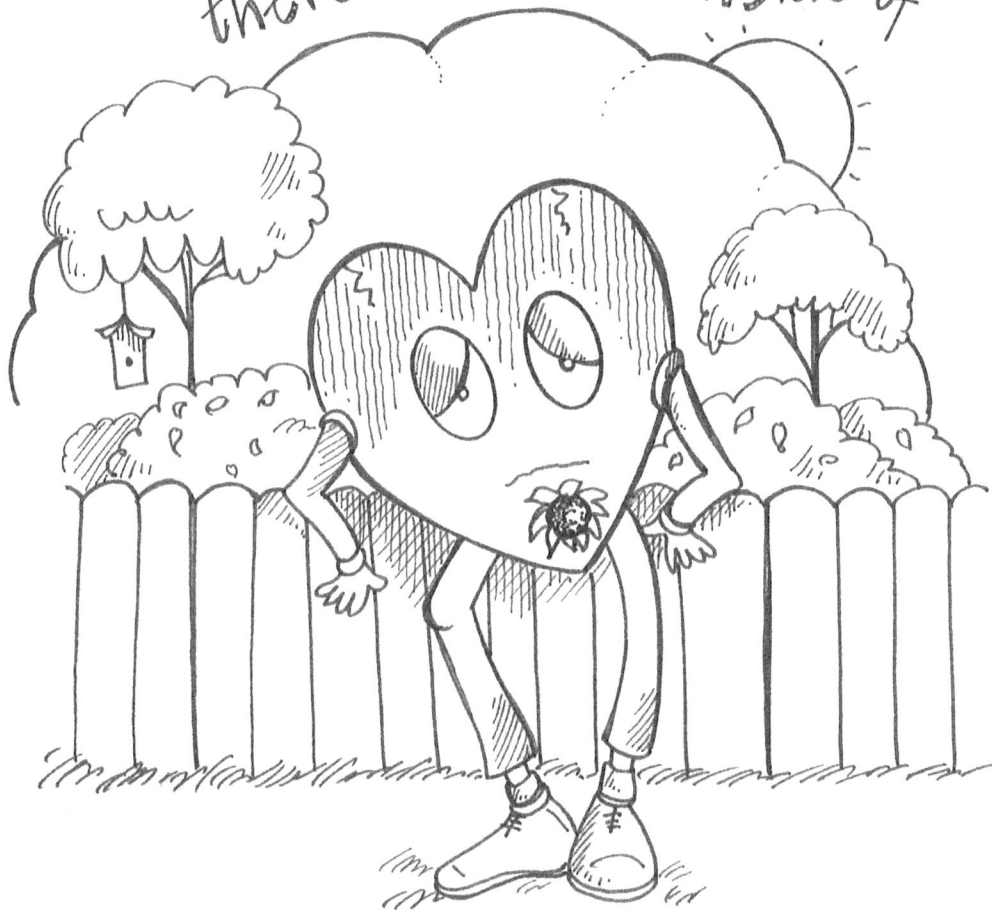

I ended up feeling that there was a hole inside of me

and that part of me was missing.

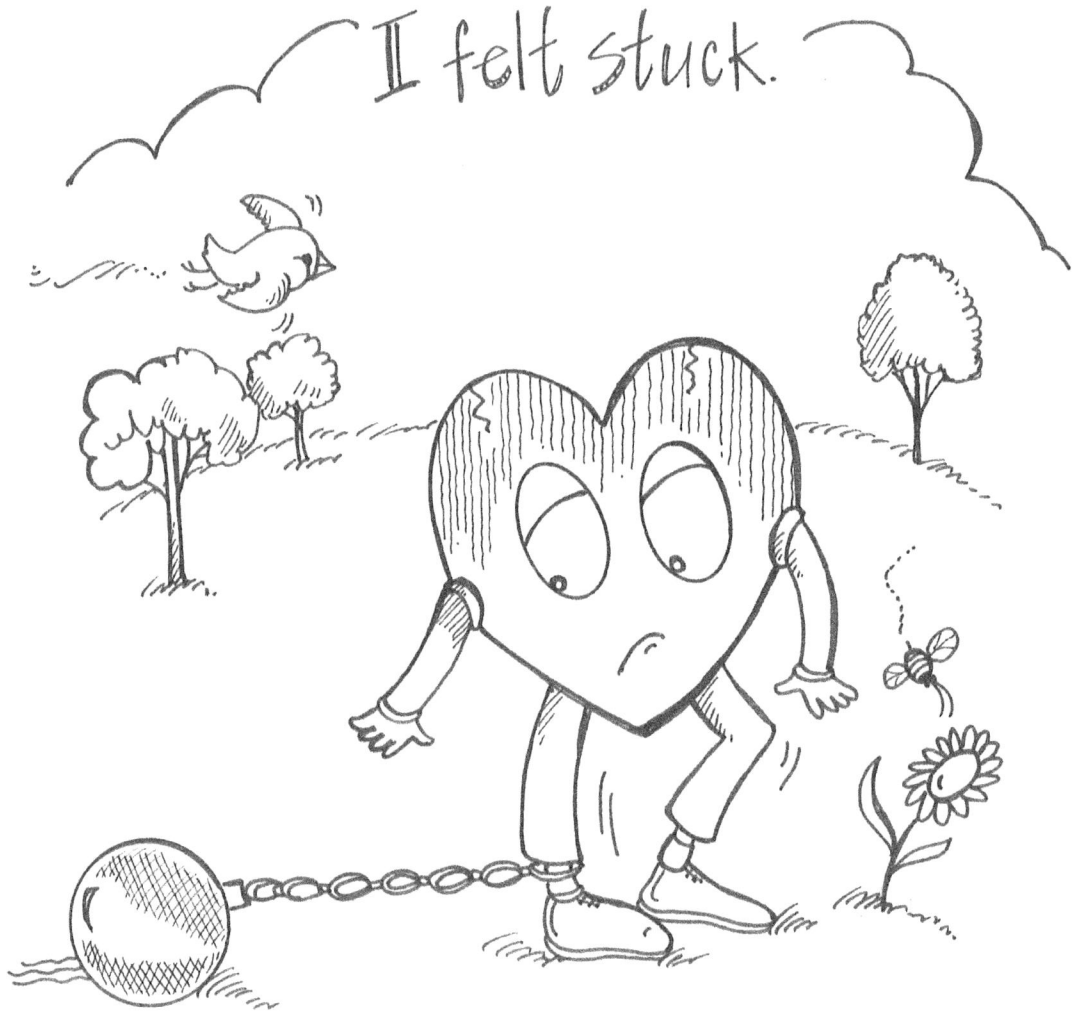

I felt stuck.

It seemed things
may not improve for me.

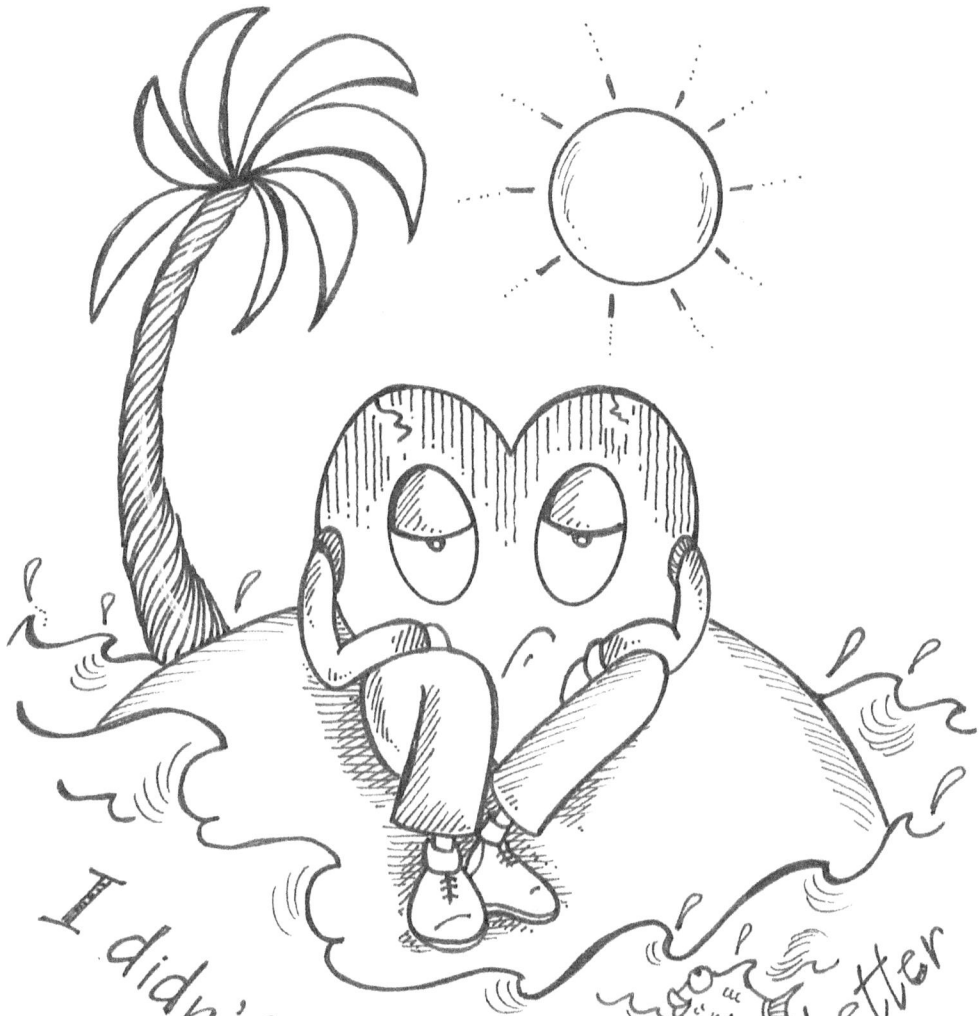

I didn't know how to get better and where to go to get help. I was afraid to be judged and criticized.

Along the way I met a
helper heart

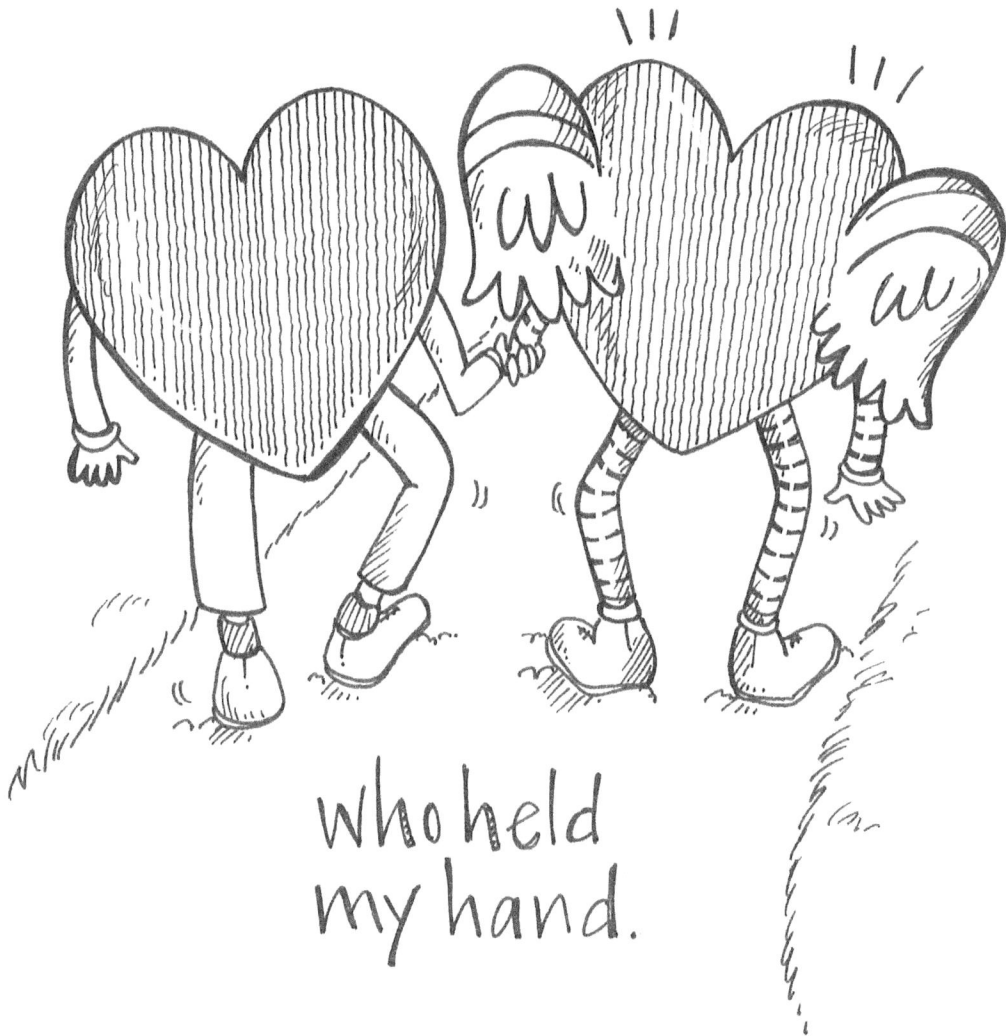

who held
my hand.

The helper heart told me
that there were

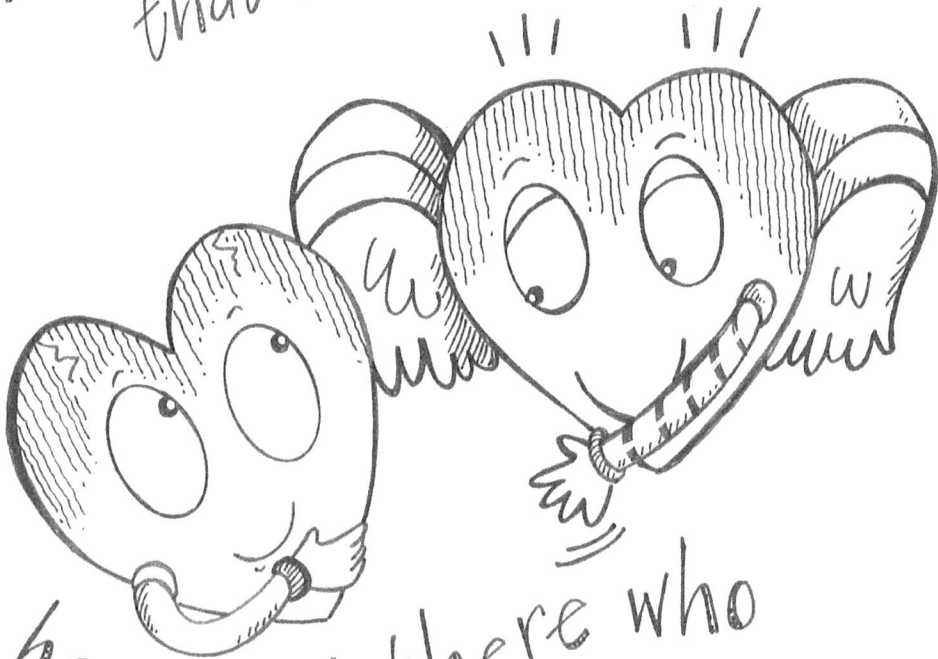

hearts out there who
were willing to help
young broken hearts
heal.

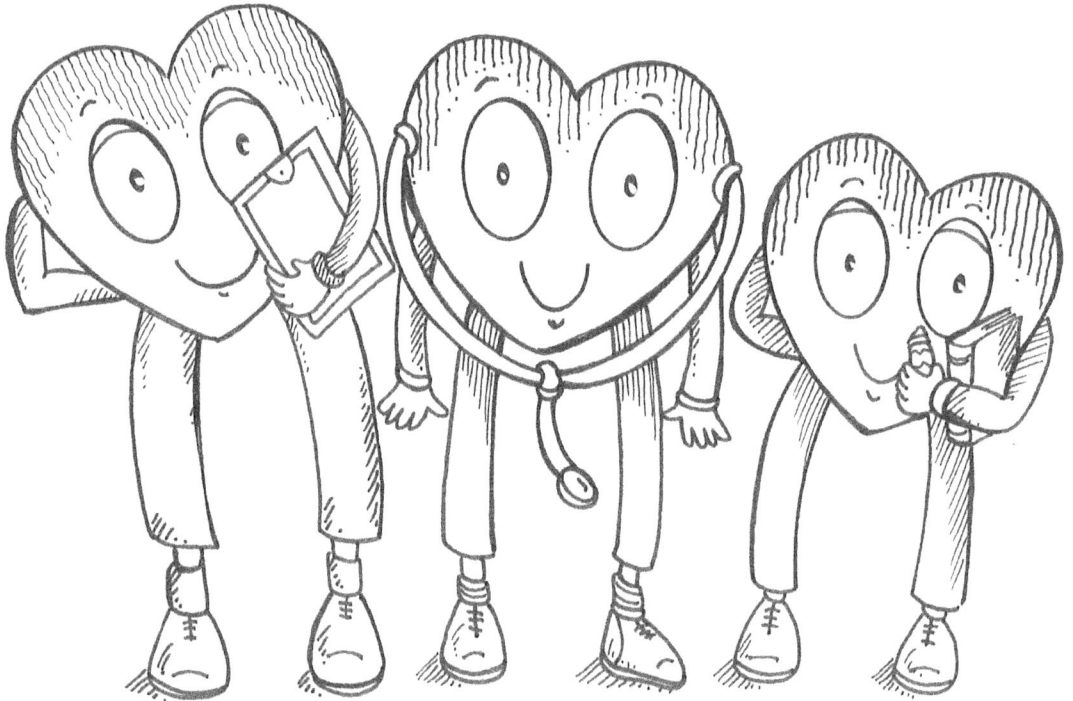

I was introduced to

counselor
hearts

doctor
hearts

teacher
hearts

and mentor hearts
amongst many others.

The helper heart taught
me that my feelings
were

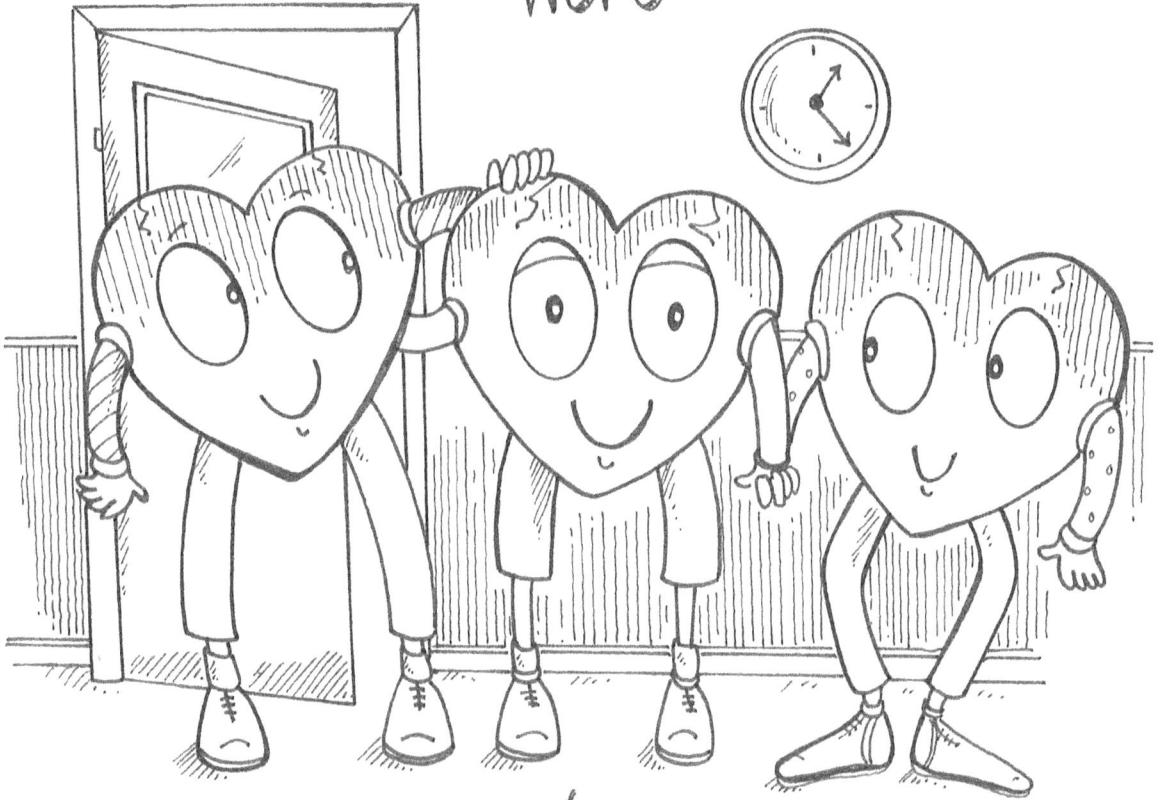

common to young
broken hearts.
I was not alone feeling this
way.

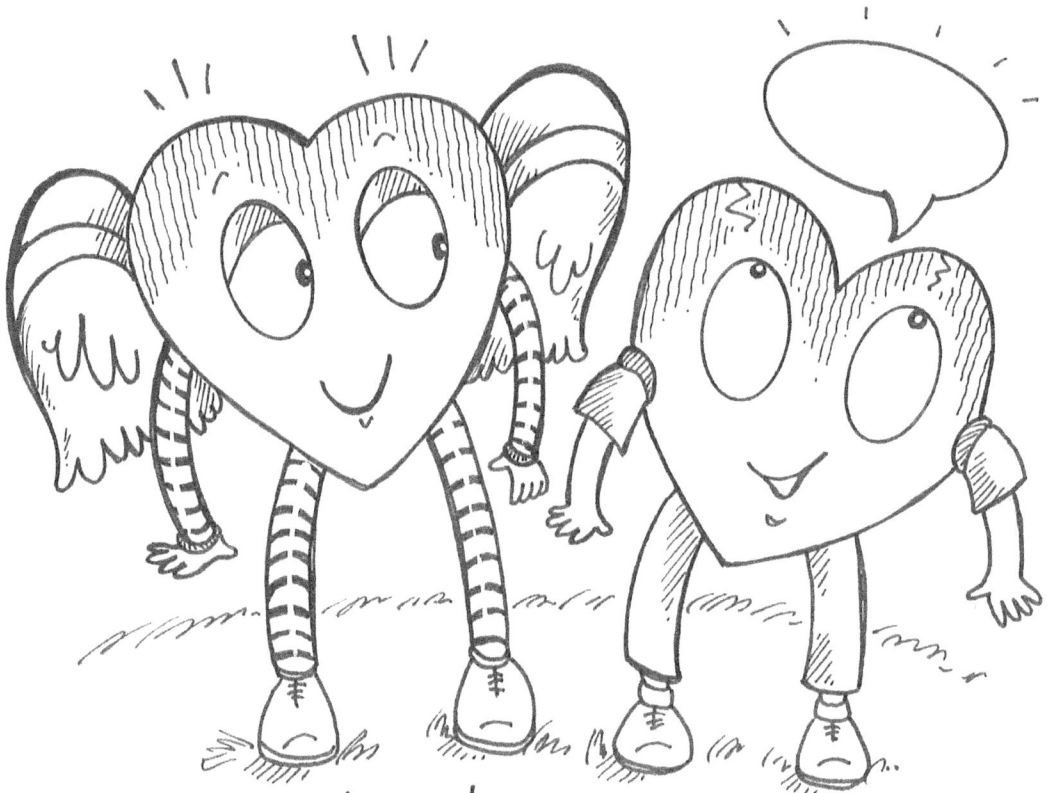

I was told that I was precious
and that I

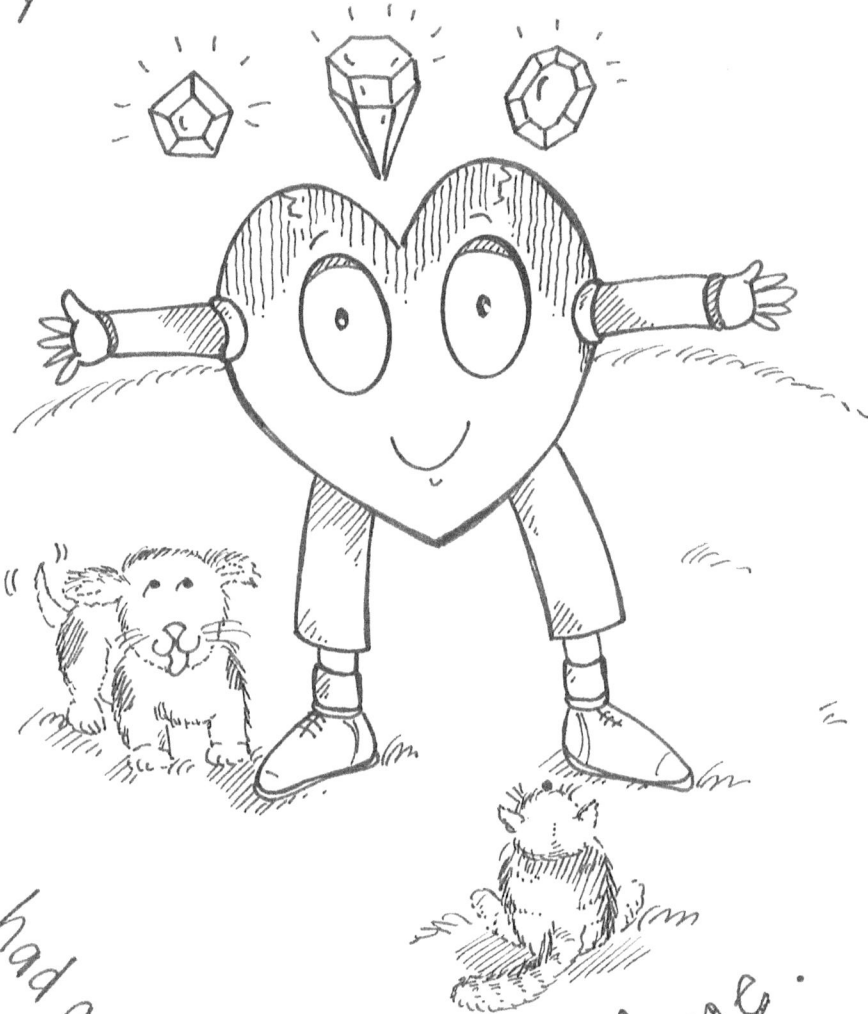

had good things inside of me.
I was worthy of being helped.

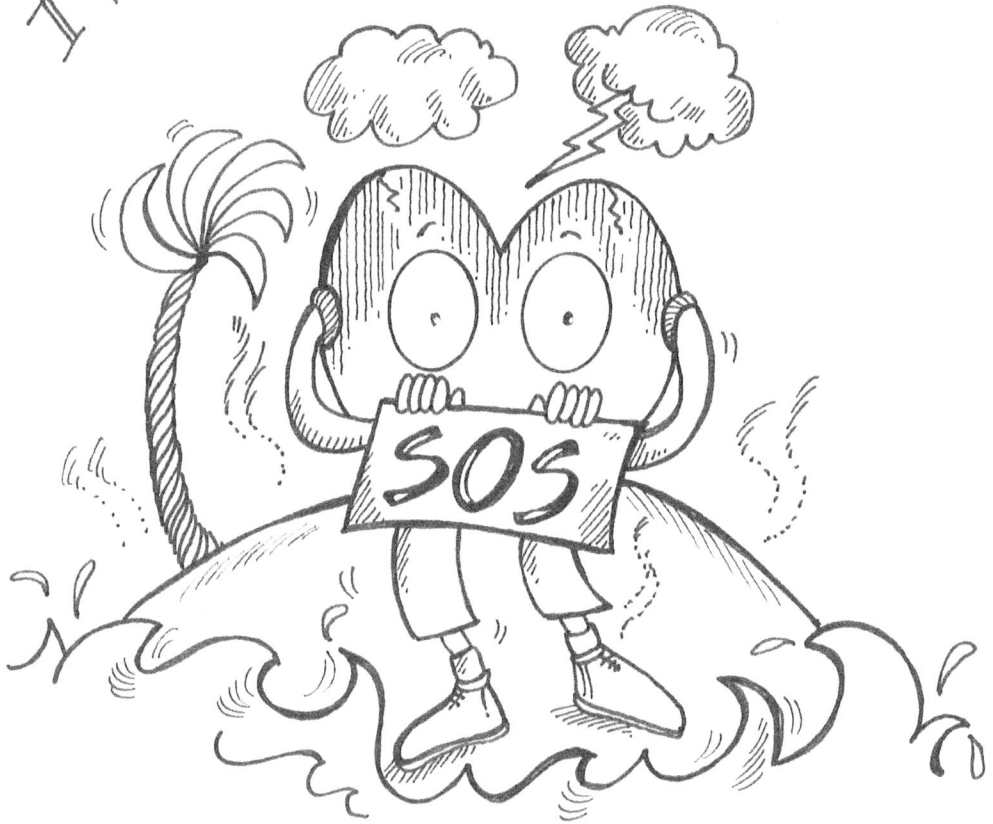

I learned to reach out when

SOS

I needed to, like when
I felt unsafe or
out of control.

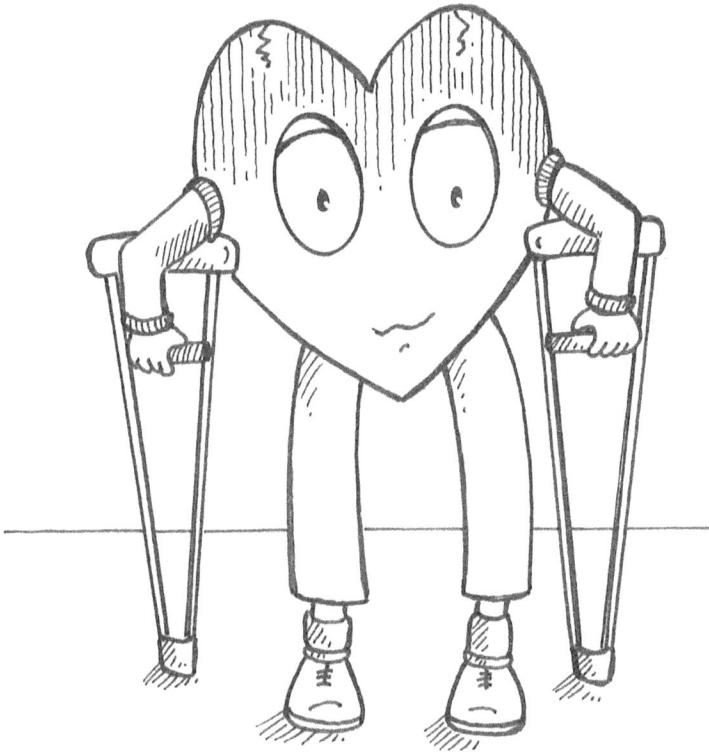

The helper heart taught me that the heart can

get better over time with the right kind of help.

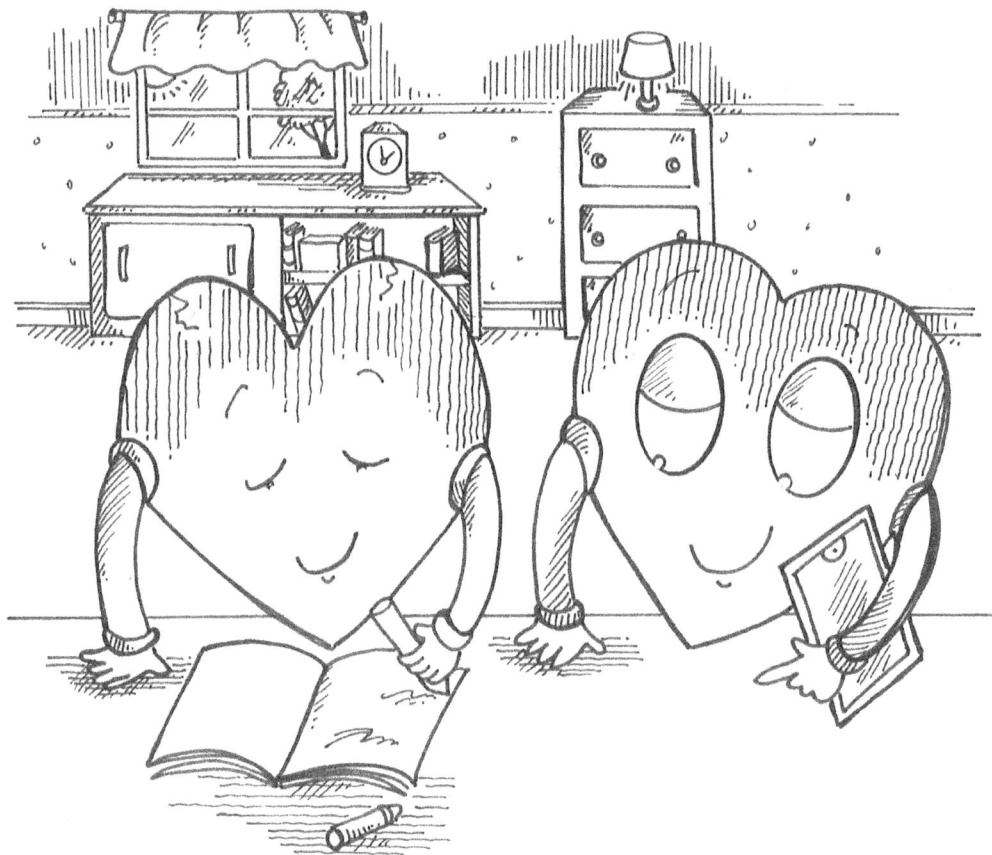

I was shown that therapy
would help me express
and understand my
feelings better.

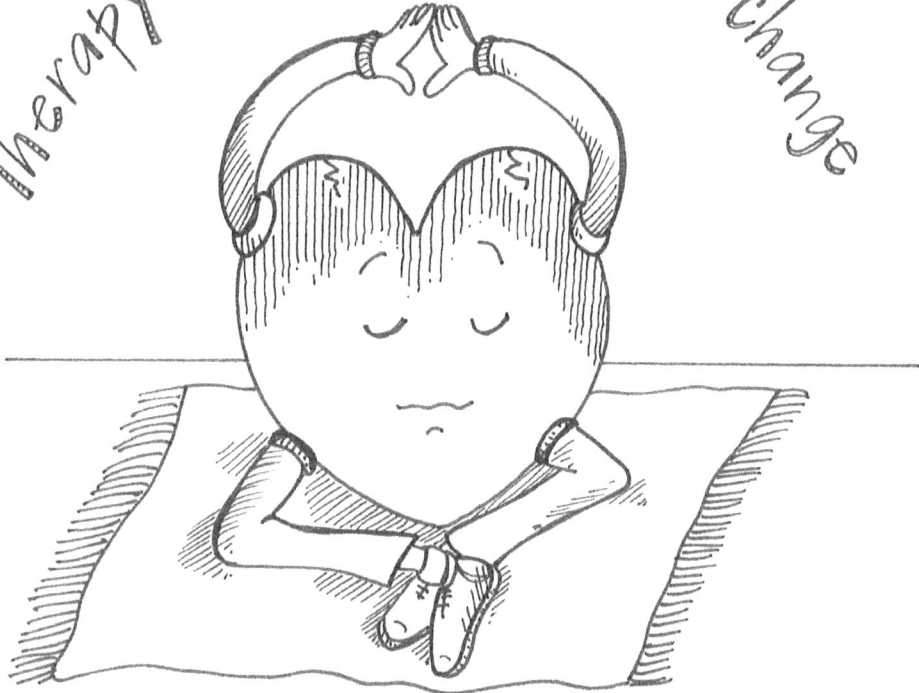

Therapy would also help me change

my behaviors
and
practice self control.

I would even be able to better understand

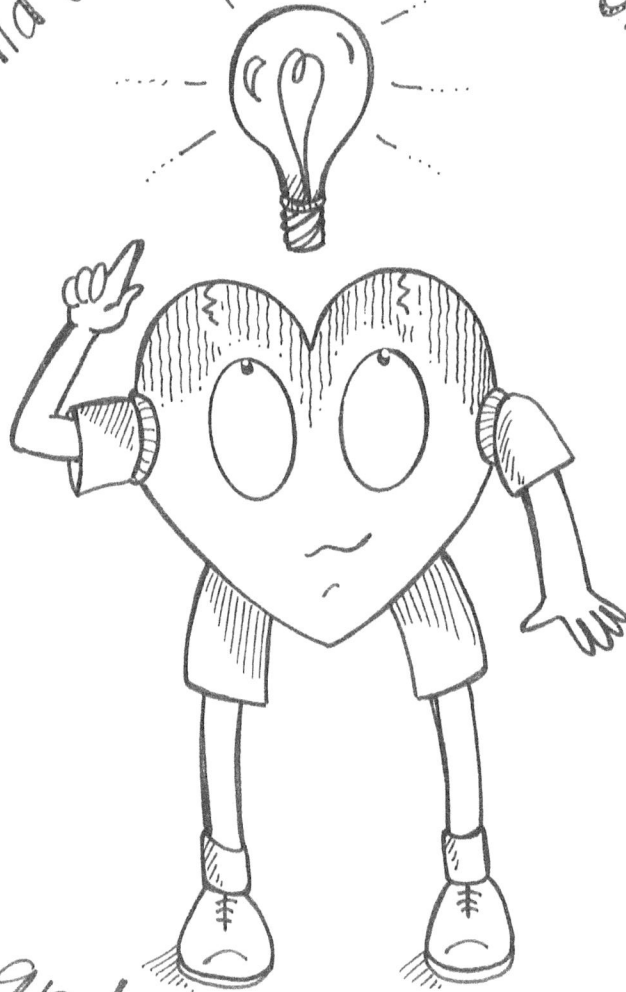

and make sense of all
the confusing things I saw.

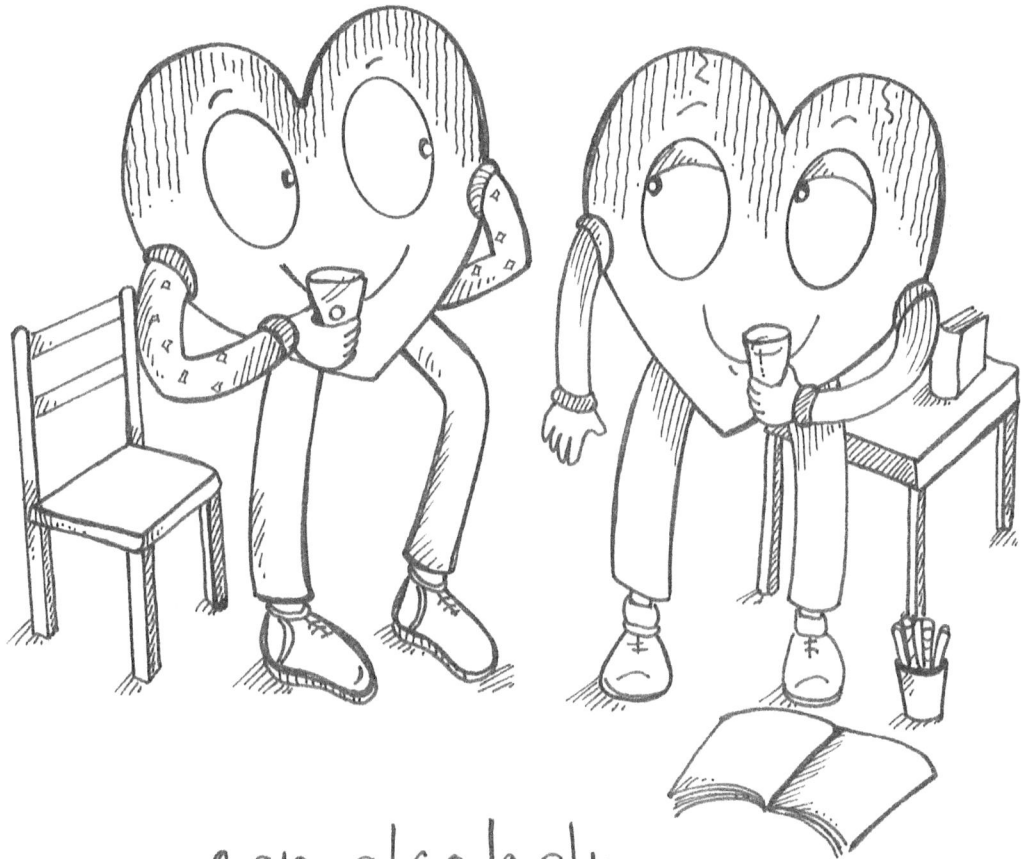

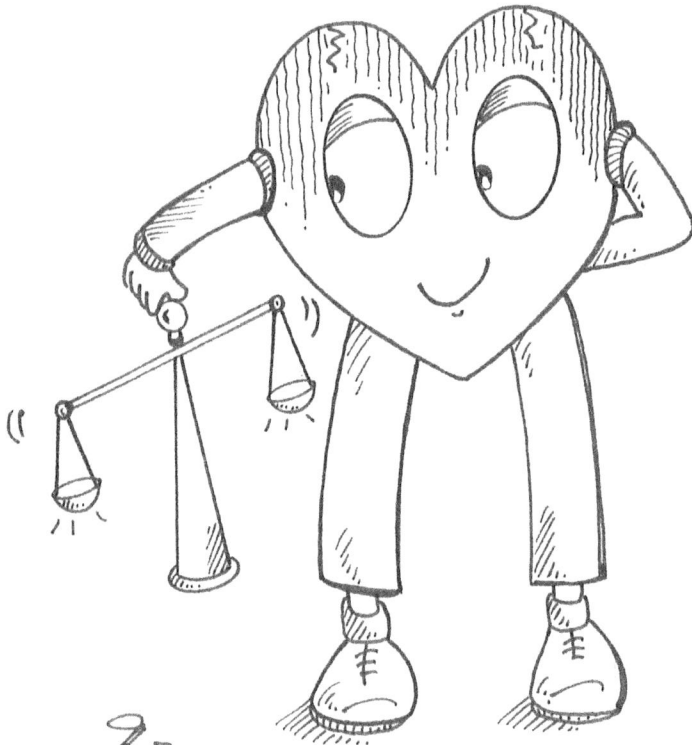

The helper heart showed me that I could receive assistance in order to have more balance and more stability in my life.

I had seen dark moments in my

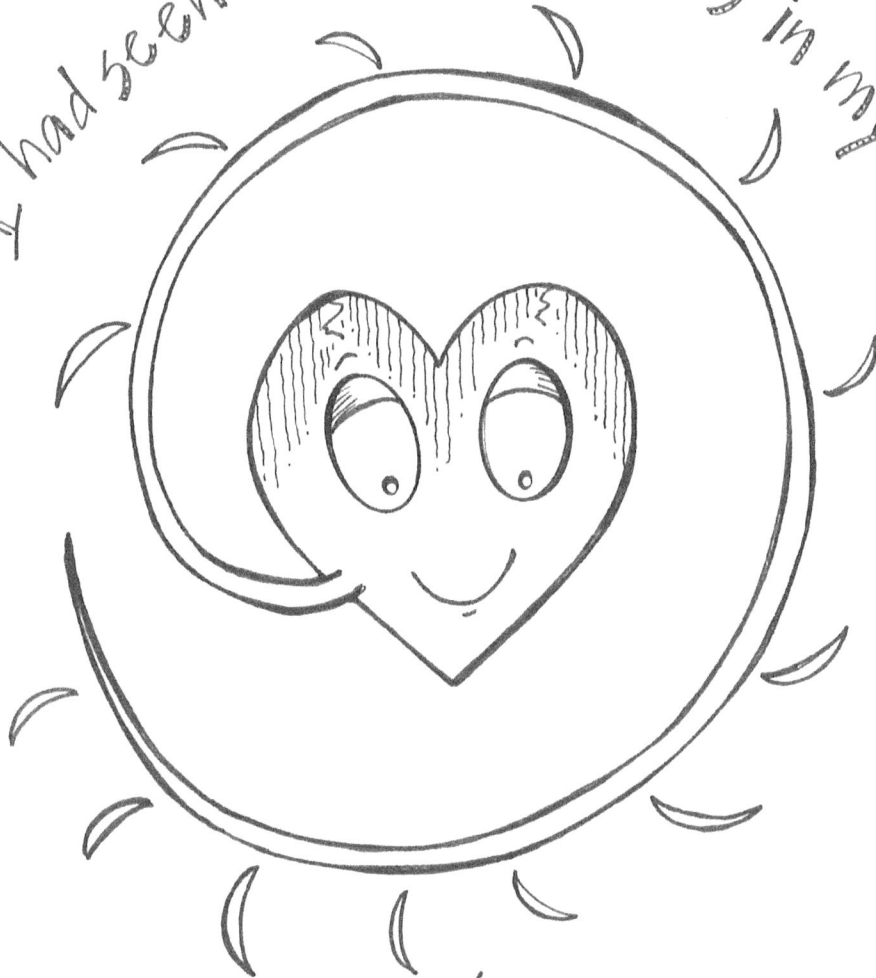

past.

I started to see a ray of hope...
a light of
understanding and healing.

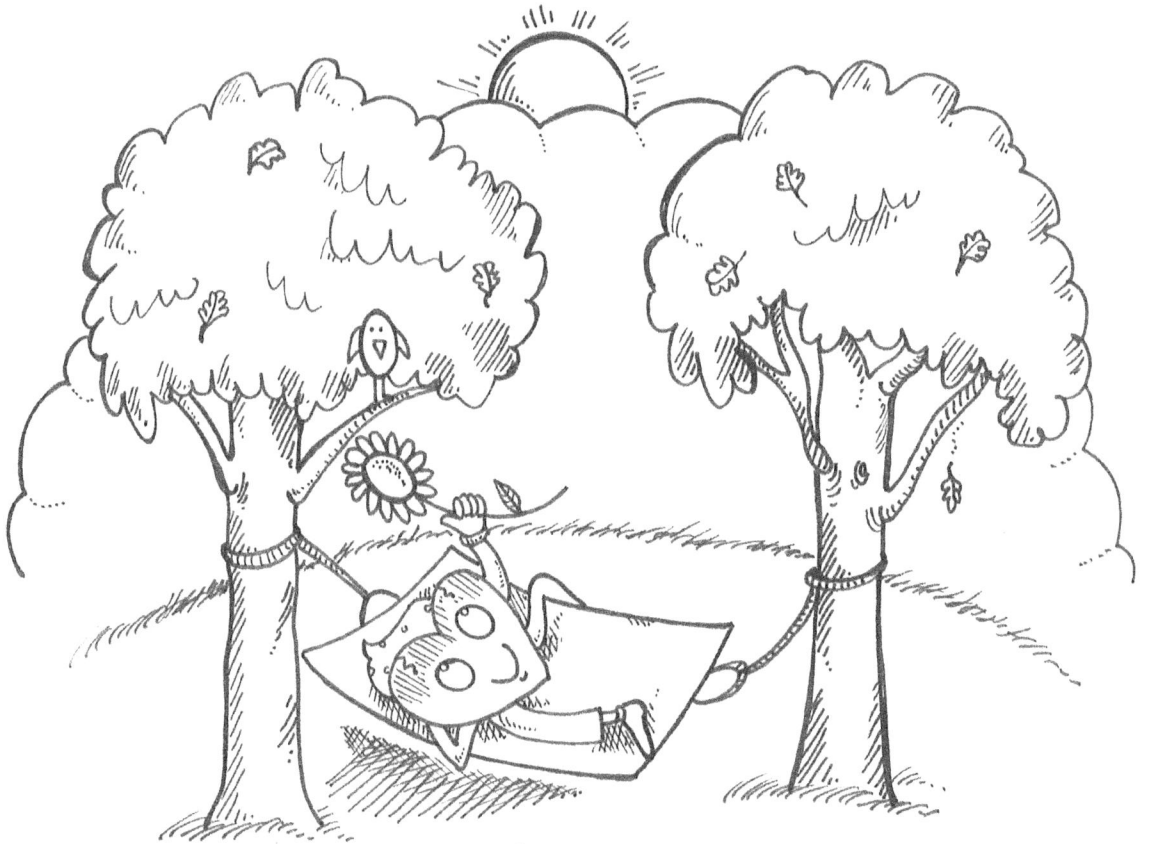

When I looked back, it felt that I had been in

survival mode at times.
I started to feel more relaxed and less tense.

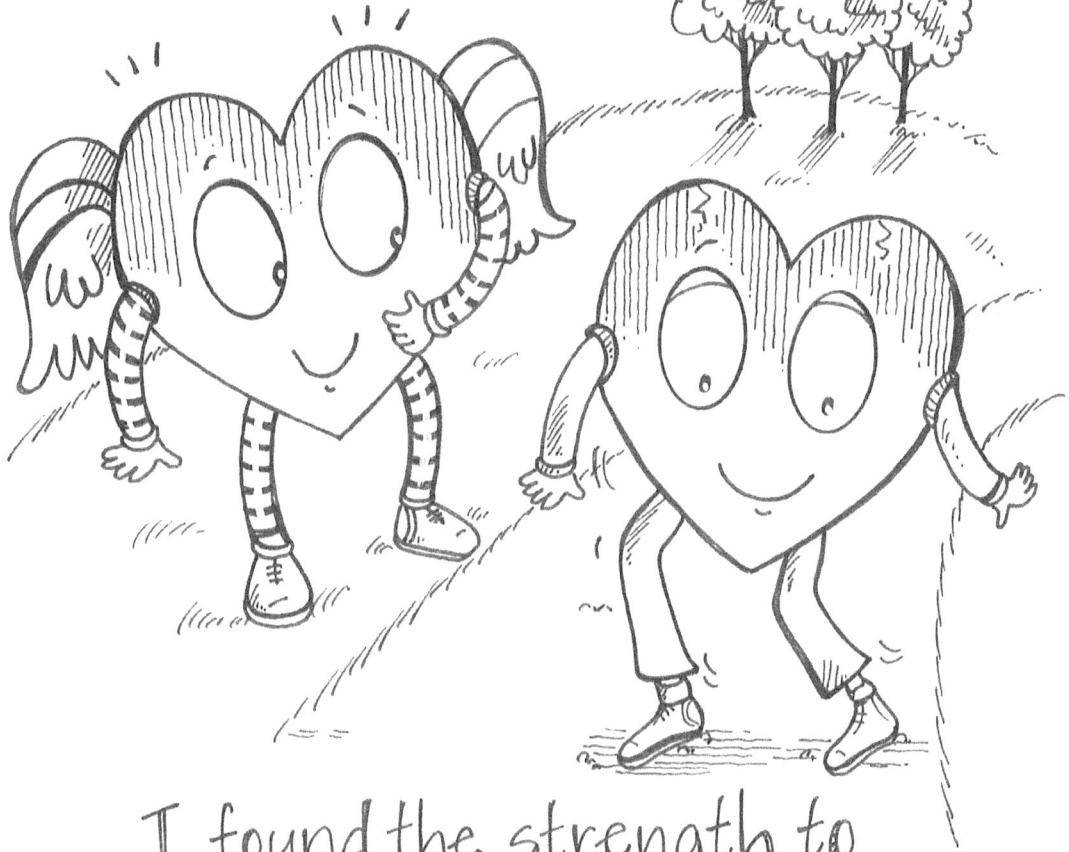

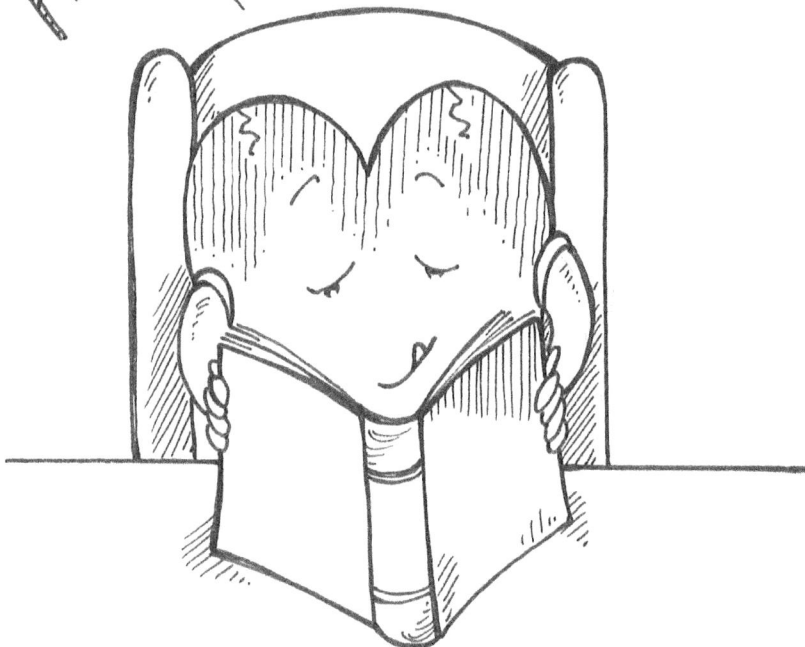

Healing takes practice

I was willing to practice
and
learn.

The helper heart told me that
I was a brave heart
who had been under
a lot of pressure.

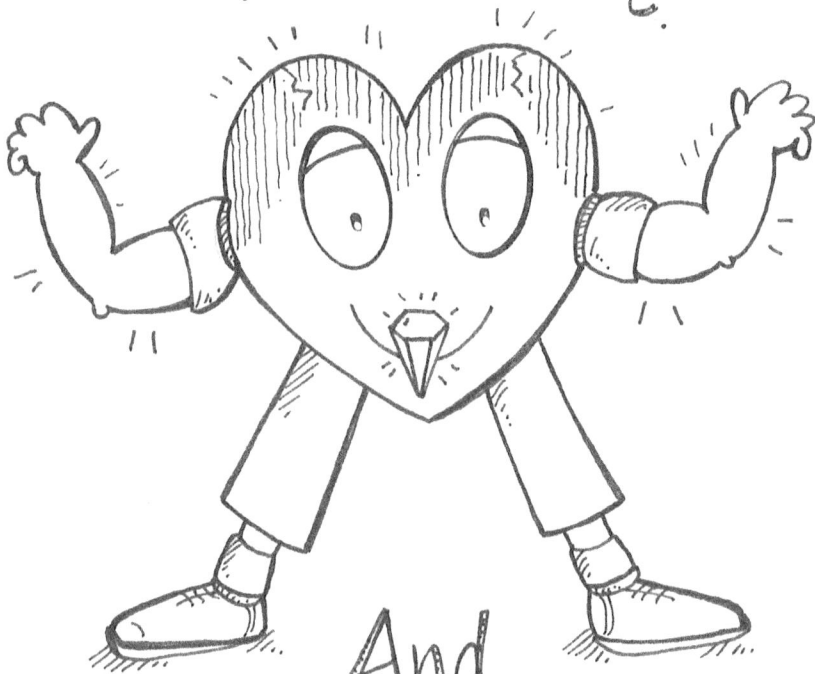

And
that a diamond was
starting to grow
inside of me.

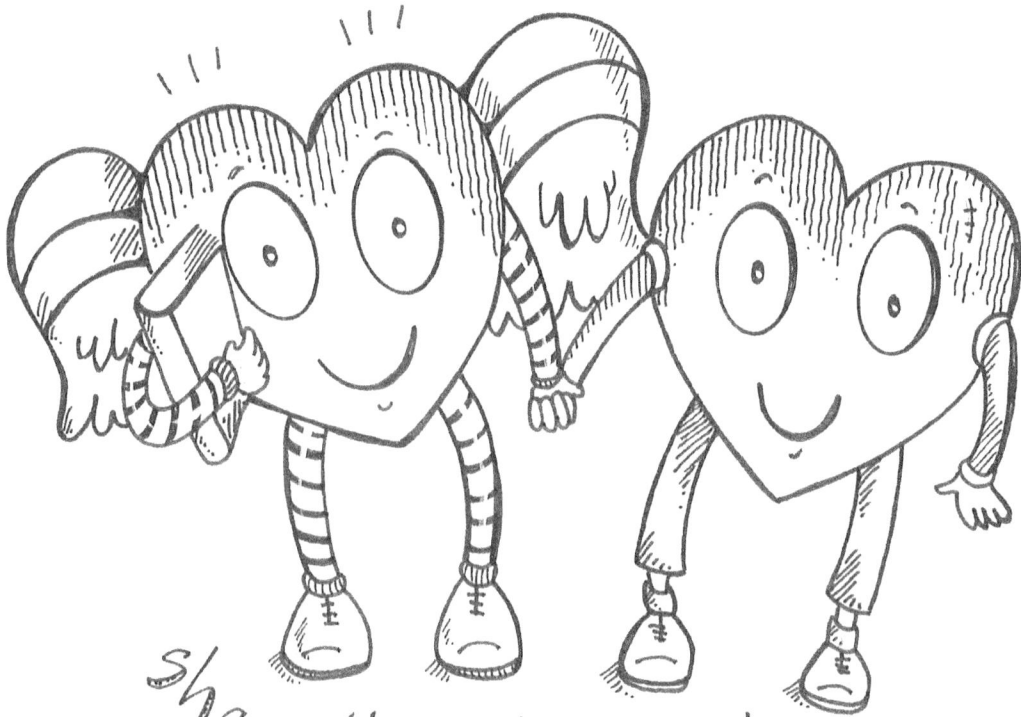

"Thank you for letting us share this story with you. We wish you the best on your healing journey."

About the author

Alexandra Schick was born and raised in France. She did her psychiatry residency at CAMC in West Virginia, and her child and adolescent psychiatry fellowship at Carilion in Virginia. She is currently practicing child and adolescent psychiatry at Highland Hospital and at Highland Psychiatric Residential Treatment Facility in Charleston WV. She is married and has two children

www.ingramcontent.com/pod-product-compliance
Lightning Source LLC
Chambersburg PA
CBHW051426200326
41520CB00023B/7378

* 9 7 8 0 6 9 2 9 7 6 9 8 2 *